MY JOURNEY

MY JOURNEY

FROM PARKINSON'S DISEASE TO DBS SURGERY

Elizabeth Larsen

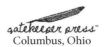
gatekeeper press™
Columbus, Ohio

My Journey: FROM PARKINSON'S DISEASE TO DBS SURGERY

Published by Gatekeeper Press
2167 Stringtown Rd, Suite 109
Columbus, OH 43123-2989
www.GatekeeperPress.com

The editorial work for this book was done by Colella Communications, LLC. Gatekeeper Press did not participate in and is not responsible for any aspect of these elements.

Library of Congress Control Number: 2021930064

ISBN (paperback): 9781662908972
eISBN: 9781662908989

TABLE OF CONTENTS

A CANDID LOOK AT PARKINSON'S DISEASE FROM A PATIENT'S POINT OF VIEW

ELIZABETH'S STORY

It's often said that you do not realize what you have until it is gone. This sentiment has never meant more to me than it did when I was diagnosed with Parkinson's disease.

The condition comes on slowly. You may realize that you trip occasionally while you're walking, you notice that small gestures are slower than they used to be, and you discover that when you're talking to people, you're not making facial expressions that you think you are. These things happened to me, but I did not think anything of them at the time. I finally went to a neurologist and he explained to me what was going on. I had to accept that I had Parkinson's disease.

This book is an overview of my life before Parkinson's disease, what it is like living with PD, and my decision regarding Deep Brain Stimulation (DBS) surgery.

If you have PD or know someone that does, this book is for you. It is a realistic look at living with PD and having DBS surgery.

DEDICATION

This book is for all my friends and family who have been with me throughout my journey so far. I love and appreciate all of you!

It is also dedicated to those of you diagnosed with Parkinson's disease.

Remember you are not alone!

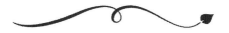

INTRODUCTION

I am not a writer by trade. I am simply a person who was diagnosed with Parkinson's disease (PD) in my 40s. This story is a true account of my journey through life, beginning with highlights prior to the Parkinson's diagnosis, then dealing with Parkinson's disease, and finally undergoing DBS surgery. I'm sharing this story with the hope that it will help others who are diagnosed with Parkinson's disease and those that are trying to decide if DBS surgery is right for them.

Although the story is true, some of the names have been changed for various reasons.

It is important to keep in mind that everyone's Parkinson's symptoms could be different, but it is still PD and still debilitating. This book was written to give you some comfort in knowing that even if your symptoms are not identical to mine, we understand each other and you are not alone.

Stay strong and keep moving!

Elizabeth Larsen

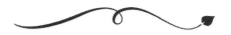

CHAPTER 1
GROWING UP

Parkinson's disease (PD) affects nearly one million people in the United States and more than six million people worldwide as of 2020. I am one of them. My name is Elizabeth (or Liz) Larsen. This is my story of my life before being diagnosed with Parkinson's disease, living with Parkinson's disease, and what I decided to do about DBS (Deep Brain Stimulation) surgery.

Prior to PD setting in, my life was active and filled with family and friends. My story began when I was born in Brooklyn, New York in January of 1964. My family at that time was made up of my parents, Bob and Marie, and my brother James. I was one of those lucky kids who, for quite a while, knew all four of my grandparents and two great-grandparents. I also had a good number of aunts, uncles, and cousins. We lived in an apartment building where all the tenants were relatives. My aunt was the landlord and my cousins Juliet and Annmarie lived above us. My dad's parents, Ronnie and Willie, lived in my building and my mom's parents, Ida and Sam, lived next door.

Although I was young, I can remember many good and not-so-good times there. I loved going to hang out at both of my grandparents' apartments. I would watch my Grandma

Ida cook or play with a china set my Grandma Ronnie kept for me at her house. Both grandmothers were very strong and independent women, which I'm sure was an influence on me. My brother James was two years younger than me and I was quite protective of him. We shared bunk beds, where I slept on top. I liked living with all our family around us, but I was a young kid who was getting spoiled. I don't know if my parents enjoyed it as much as I did.

In 1970, when I was six, my parents, like many others, moved the family to Staten Island, New York, which was close to the city but felt like the suburbs. We ended up in an area called Great Kills. My sister Kristine was born in 1971 and three years later, my brother Matthew arrived. Great Kills was a good place to grow up, with lots of nice families with kids, tree-lined streets, and beautiful houses. It was safe to walk anywhere. We lived only four blocks away from my parents' best friends and cousins, Carmine and Rosemary. These are my Romano cousins from my mom's side of the family. They have three daughters – Marianne, Christine, and Danielle. Our families were remarkably close then and still are today.

We are all fans of the movie The Wizard of Oz, and it has always been my favorite. One of my fondest memories is of all of us watching The Wizard of Oz together when we were young. There is also one quote about the film that I associate with my journey: "It's not where you go, it's who you meet along the way." I was fortunate to have many supportive family members and friends throughout my life. They have helped me grow, have taught me so much, and have been an integral part of my story through the years – sometimes in ways I never could have imagined.

My parents believed in taking one vacation each year with us children and one without. For a few summers, James and I would spend a week at my Aunt Bea's house in Bayville, Long Island. She lived four houses from the beach in a homey yet beautiful house. We did crafts, spent time at the beach, and had all kinds of fun that brought James and me even closer as we grew up.

As a preteen, I used to get bored, so of course I would watch TV. This led to my love of watching sports, especially football. When my dad was not busy, I would watch the New York Giants football games with him. Over the years, I continued to connect with people through sports and fantasy football, both before and after PD.

While I was growing up, I remember my mother decorating and baking for every holiday. When I was an adult, I asked her why she still decorated the house even though we were not children anymore. She said, "I decorate because I enjoy it. I don't only do it for you. When I do not like it anymore, then I will not do it." That day never came. She decorated until she died at age 65 and I follow her advice. No matter how sick I am or how hard decorating may be, as long as I continue to enjoy it, I will do it.

My family went through a rough time from 1985 to 1989, when both of my mom's parents and my brother James died. James had a rare kidney condition that probably stemmed from having a virus as a baby, but the damage it did was not detected until he was in fourth or fifth grade. He had a kidney transplant in 1983 and fought a constant battle against his body rejecting it. He finished high school, graduating in a wheelchair, and lived until 1988, when he developed pneumonia and was hospitalized. We had always been very close siblings and when

I went to visit him there for the last time, just before he passed away, I intuitively knew something was wrong. I urged the rest of the family to visit as soon as they could and they did. I had to work and never got to see him again. This changed my work/life balance attitude for the rest of my career.

While my brother was growing up and going through his illness, my mother and father each dealt with it and supported him in different ways. My mother went to college to learn about biology and now that I think about it, perhaps the way she educated herself about what my brother had would later influence the way I handled my own health issues. My dad, meanwhile, did renovations to the house to make things more accommodating for James and his wheelchair and help him however possible. In later years, that same sense of familial support would be a lifeline for me, as well.

The loss of my mother's parents and James put a lot of stress on all of us. The saying that bad things, particularly people dying, happen in threes rang true for me during those years. It would happen again between 2006 and 2011, when I lost both of my parents as well as my grandmother. When my father and my Grandma Ronnie died, I had to make the painful decision to take each of them off the machines that were helping them breathe.

My parents died before my grandmother, which left me responsible for her. I loved her, but she did not live in the best area of Brooklyn. I had to go there every weekend with groceries and it stressed me out. Eventually, I moved her to a nursing home in Staten Island where she lived until she passed away in 2011, and I am grateful she was not alone. My Parkinson's symptoms were starting around this time, but I ignored them because I felt I did not have time to deal with my problems. My grandmother needed me and that came at the expense of my own health.

Some may wonder whether my Parkinson's was due to genetics and I don't know the answer. Looking back, I remember my grandmother's hands shaking to some extent, but it could be attributed to her age at the time. And when my mother died in 2006, after more than forty years of marriage, my father had a terrible time dealing with it. He had various health issues, too, and it wasn't until he lost a lot of weight and changed some medications that I recall his hands trembling at times. But it could have been attributed to the medicines and he passed away soon after.

For a long time, my sister and her family lived in Staten Island. I was close to them, particularly to my nephew Peter. He would sleep over at my house, where we would hang out or I would take him to the zoo, circus, or movies. Around 2015, they moved upstate and I was able to visit them there until my Parkinson's got so bad that it was difficult to drive.

My brother and his family, including his twins Kyla and Anthony, live in Florida. I stay in touch with them using FaceTime and would try to visit whenever I could, but that became harder as my Parkinson's got worse.

Shortly after my parents and Grandma Ronnie died, my PD began taking over. Annmarie, her husband Tommie, Carmine, Rosemary, and their families helped me through that difficult time. My family knew I had PD even before I could admit it. They have all seen PD make me weak, assisted me when I could not walk on my own, and watched me bounce back from DBS surgery. Their contributions of time and donations helped build my non-profit company and as a result, helped build my spirit, as well. I attribute their constant support to the strong bond we all had growing up.

In addition to my family members, I have especially close relationships with three girlfriends – Dorothea, Erin, and Greta, who was my papergirl. They are some of the most important people in my life and we have been friends for more than forty years! In 1991, the girls were getting together around Christmastime to have champagne and open presents. Since I was having a tough year, they invited me to cheer me up. This was our first "Girls Christmas." We are still having this annual get-together and it's the best day of the year. There is champagne, brie, lots of presents, and stockings filled with surprises. I love these girls as if they were sisters. They would also turn out to be the ones to eventually help me make one of the biggest decisions of my life.

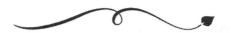

CHAPTER 2
MARRIAGE IS NOT FOR EVERYONE

At the age of fourteen, I started dating my first boyfriend. He played baseball and softball and I was always at his games, keeping score. For years, we would hang out with a large group of friends, get a keg or cases of beer, and head to the woods, park, or beach where we listened to music, laughed, and drank. As we got older, we started going to neighborhood bars and in the summer, we would go down to the New Jersey Shore. There were so many good times, and these are friends that remain by my side today.

My first marriage was to my childhood sweetheart in 1989. It was February, not even a year after my brother died. The marriage did not last long, but to this day, the wedding was the best party I ever threw. We had a big reception, with more than 200 guests and a DJ from the Jersey shore. The highlights of the wedding were not the first dance or the cake cutting, but rather when we began to dance to Eric Clapton's song, "Wonderful Tonight." All our friends started singing in their loudest voices. The best part, though, was when we were up on people's shoulders, singing Meatloaf's "Paradise by the Dashboard Lights," the groom wearing no shirt and me wearing sunglasses. The dance floor was packed the entire night and everybody was having the time of their lives. Although the marriage did not last, my ex-husband and I have circled back to being friends. He helped me start my golf outing fundraiser. He is on the board of my company and supports me in my fight against PD.

Many of the friends who attended our wedding also still support me in my efforts to raise donations for Parkinson's research and assist me when I'm having a hard time. In 2019, several of the guys played in an over-50 softball league. Whenever I could, I went to the games even though walking on the grass was difficult. My nephew Matty would keep score and we would share many laughs while I sat with him. It felt good to be out and together with people, and one of the guys would help me to my car afterward. It was at one of these games that my friend Joe advised me that if I were a candidate, I should have the DBS surgery. He was someone I trusted, so it meant a lot when he said this.

My second marriage came with a bit more resistance from those around me. I can be very hardheaded sometimes and against the advice of many people, I got involved with a friend's brother. He had two young boys, Mike and Alex. Whenever we were alone or with the boys, things were great, but as soon as decisions needed to be made or life got hard, it sucked. His tendency to lie only made things worse, but my stubbornness got the better of me. I did not want to be alone, so I married him.

During this relationship, when I was thirty-five, I found out I could not have children. One of my life philosophies is, "Everything happens for a reason." I truly feel this applies to my second marriage and fully believe I was meant to be the boys' stepmom. Even though their father and I have been divorced for years, Mike and Alex remain an important part of my life. They have both grown into wonderful young men that I am proud of and love as if they were my own. Mike, too, would eventually play a big part in helping me get through the first DBS surgery.

My biggest fear used to be living alone. As it turns out, living on my own is pretty good and I can handle it much better than I thought. Now my biggest fear is living with Parkinson's disease.

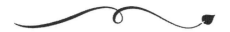

CHAPTER 3
WORK/LIFE BALANCE

Before my Parkinson's disease diagnosis, I led an active lifestyle. I tried to have something to do every weekend and went out during the week after work as much as I could.

From 1987 through 2019, I worked in Manhattan in various jobs. The two jobs I held the longest and where I made the most friends were at CMR, a media research company, and most recently at Moody's, a credit rating agency. My friends from CMR were supportive when my mother died. It was unexpected and my family was devastated, but my colleagues stood by me.

My Parkinson's started around the end of my tenure at CMR. I started working at Moody's about fifteen months after leaving CMR and felt good when I first started the new job. I was able to take handwritten notes, commuting to Manhattan was not an issue, my walking was okay, and the left side tremors were minimal.

However, my health steadily declined throughout my time at Moody's. My shaking worsened and taking notes became difficult. Initially, I was able to walk pretty well by following the blocks in the sidewalk and listening to music, but eventually walking became harder as my balance grew worse. I still followed those blocks in the pavement and listened to music, but could no longer talk to anyone while I was walking. I had problems at the top of staircases and in doorways and began to trip and fall due to the smallest inconsistencies in the sidewalk. After I fell at least six to eight times, I eventually stopped walking outside to get lunch and stayed in the building to go to the cafeteria.

Even staying indoors could be challenging. Our office was at 1 World Trade Center on a newly built-out floor and on either side of the main hallway, there were inclines that were hard to see. Going to a meeting one day, I tripped and fell. Afterward, I helped devise a way to make it easier to notice the incline and they switched the rug color for those two spots. I also participated on the first-ever Disability Panel.

There was a reason I was working at Moody's during this stage of my illness. It was the people. I had many friends who helped me and never made me feel bad if I were having a hard time or could not do something. My friend Lou lived near me, so when I came to the office, he would try to leave at the same time I did so we could commute home together. He would walk me to my car, drive it to my house, and then walk to his own house. Other friends would bring me lunch so I did not have to walk to the cafeteria.

My closest friend at work was my boss, Matt. We worked out a flexible schedule so that, even though my Parkinson's was getting worse, I could still work and be productive. He talked me off the ledge many times and gave me helpful advice when I needed it. He is no longer at Moody's, but we remain close friends.

I have local friends and neighbors that support me, as well. One neighbor brings in my garbage pails each week. It is incredible how helpful that one small gesture is when you are struggling to simply walk. Kristin is another friend who used to be my neighbor and she is the reason why I moved onto the block where I live. Her daughter Hannah, who I consider my niece, would come over to hang out and talk. Sometimes her boyfriend or brothers would also come to hang out or help me, which always cheered me up. Whenever I was able, I would also walk over to their house for dinner and drinks. It was good for me to get out. Unfortunately, they recently had to move and no longer live nearby.

I'm close to other neighbors, Ginny and Mike, who frequently invite me over for a dice game called Bones. We usually play with Fran and Joe plus a few other friends every weekend. As I write this book, we are in the middle of a pandemic, which jarred our in-person games to a halt. Luckily, during the quarantine, we figured out a way to play the game virtually. This was a major positive for me, since I live on my own and talk to myself more than I should. I enjoy their friendship and company, whether it is face-to-face or over my computer screen.

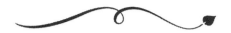

CHAPTER 4
THE SYMPTOMS BEGIN

In 2013, at a birthday party for Greta, I was helping to clean up but moving very slowly. My friend Joanne came up to me and asked what the hell was going on. She emotionally told me that I could not continue to live like this. She was right. I finally had to admit that I had Parkinson's disease. That was the scariest reality I had to face – even harder than telling my grandmother that her only child, my father, had died. No one wants to be sick with a disease that has no cure. I cried, had a pity party, and then picked myself up and realized I had to start dealing with this. It was not a death sentence, but it was going to mean a change in my lifestyle.

Once I accepted the diagnosis, I found myself looking back on how it started. I thought about how the symptoms came on slowly, over time. I had been occasionally tripping and stubbing my foot as I walked. This may not seem like a big deal, but it started happening often enough that I noticed and was bothered by it. My left hand was shaking – again, not a lot, but enough to interfere with my day-to-day life. I would hide my hand in meetings at work so people would not see it shaking. My left side was stiff and my left arm became virtually immobile as I walked. My upper lip was trembling all the time. My movements were slowing down and it was becoming obvious.

As these symptoms grew increasingly worse, I met with several doctors to get them checked out. One doctor gave me a test that required poking me with a thin needle. I don't remember the name of the test, but I do remember the result was normal – meaning we still did not know the cause of the shaking. Then I went to my regular doctor, who recommended I see a neurologist. This doctor ran several tests and MRIs and watched me move. He ultimately observed that I was not moving my left arm much while I walked, and I admitted I hardly ever did. I realized he was trying to determine if I had Parkinson's disease. He also made me aware of some herniated discs in my neck that were impacting my left side.

Unfortunately, I found it difficult to listen to advice from this neurologist due to his terrible bedside manner. Several people that I know went to him, as well, and said the same thing. My cousin came with me when I was receiving my test results and agreed this doctor had a poor approach to handling patients. That is a shame because as it turns out, he was right about my diagnosis but I became so upset talking to him that I ignored what he said about Parkinson's and only focused on the herniated discs. I lost about one or two years of treating my PD symptoms as a result.

No matter how hard it is to hear the PD diagnosis, it is better to accept it and start dealing with it rather than stick your head in the sand and hope it gets better. Before I was diagnosed with PD, I remember thinking that if a doctor could just get my walking straightened out, then I could handle the shaking. Little did I know that my walking would get much worse before there was any chance of improvement. I ultimately began shuffling and my gait was freezing.

At first, I tried to use physical therapy to help with my neck issues rather than facing the possibility of having Parkinson's disease. A few months earlier, I had gone to a physical therapist named Vinny Puccio for a problem with my knee. He was close by my house and a great guy. I went back to him with the MRI results for my neck and we came up with a plan. Over time, physical therapy helped with the pain and stiffness in my neck, using a combination of massage, stimulation, and exercise.

Fortunately, since exercise is one of the best ways to manage PD symptoms, physical therapy was probably helping me fight the symptoms even before I was willing to accept the diagnosis. I enjoy exercising and liked going to PT, so I figured it was not so bad. I could manage that. The only problem was that the shaking in my left hand did not improve nor did the walking issues.

Since my left hand continued to shake, despite the physical therapy, I decided it was time to get a second opinion and go to a different neurologist. Vinny recommended Dr. Igor Stiler, who was much better than the previous neurologist I had seen. At my first appointment, I mentioned to him that the shaking in my left side subsided whenever I relaxed and had a glass of wine. He immediately diagnosed me with essential tremors, or ET, which is a neurological medical condition characterized by involuntary rhythmic contractions and relaxations, or twitching movements, of certain muscle groups in one or more body parts. Its cause is unknown and it is typically symmetrical, most often affecting the arms, hands, or fingers and sometimes head, vocal cords, or other body parts. It is also sometimes confused with Parkinson's disease.

Dr. Stiler and I developed a new approach to managing my symptoms. This included two medications, Propranolol and Primidone, as well as continuing physical therapy. This new plan did allow me to somewhat manage my left side tremors, but my troubles with walking intensified and new PD symptoms were starting to set in – even some that I did not realize were happening.

One of the best things I did while experiencing all these health issues was to visit a podiatrist, Dr. Michael Scotto. I figured since I was not walking properly, I should get my feet checked. I learned that continuously walking incorrectly could throw off other things, also. My right foot tends to develop a painful callus on the bottom because I lean more to that side. I also have a bunion and bad hammer toe that are unrelated to PD. I inherited these bothersome traits from my Grandma Ida. Over time, this doctor would become a friend and one of my most trusted advisors. I am still going to him today.

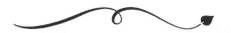

CHAPTER 5
IT IS PARKINSON'S DISEASE

From the time Dr. Stiler told me I had essential tremors, I suspected he knew I could also have Parkinson's disease. He also realized I had to accept this in my own time; otherwise, I would have walked out on him like I did my first neurologist. He needed to gain my trust and show me facts. I went for more MRIs, continued to exercise, and did everything I could to try and prove I did not have PD. And even though I would not admit it, it was still taking over my body. I fell several times and everyday chores were getting harder to do. There were many other Parkinson's-related issues going on, yet I was in full denial.

At the same time, my colleagues were beginning to take notice of my worsening symptoms. For years, I met daily with an intelligent and outspoken manager with whom I very much enjoyed working. During those meetings, he began questioning if I understood what he was talking about. This happened almost every day. I could not figure out why he was asking this, so I made a conscious effort to convey my understanding of conversations through more vivid facial expressions. Eventually, other people started making similar comments. As it turned out, unbeknownst to me, I was not making facial expressions when I spoke or listened to other people. I knew this was a symptom of Parkinson's disease. I explained what was going on to my doctor and asked him how we could discover if I had PD or not. I was still holding out hope that it was only essential tremors.

To determine whether I had Parkinson's, I had to begin taking medications to see if they helped my symptoms. I started on a combination of older but more reliable PD drugs called Ropinirole and Azilect, with a low dosage of each. This is a common combination of medicines for Parkinson's. Both the good news and the bad news was that the medicine started to work. This was good news because it helped me feel better. It was also bad news because it confirmed I had Parkinson's disease instead of essential tremors alone, as I was hoping.

I did not want to admit it, but I had to. It was time to face reality and start moving forward so I could fight this. I have Parkinson's disease. Admitting that was one of the hardest things I have ever had to do.

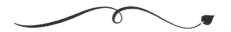

CHAPTER 6
THE INITIAL PLAN AND LIVING
WITH PD

Once I was able to accept that fact that I had Parkinson's disease, I met with my doctor and went over the options for managing the symptoms. Basically, there are two choices: medications and Deep Brain Stimulation (DBS) surgery. I had to start with the medications to see how they worked before considering surgery. The doctor also had to consider my essential tremors because I was already taking medications for those.

Parkinson's impacts everyone differently, which makes deciding which medicines to take and the dosage a constant game of trial and error. It took a while, but we eventually figured it out. Initially, I was prescribed four different medications, which amounted to nine pills daily. To this day, I am still on the same combination of medications and have come to accept them, because I now understand the side effects and how each medication impacts me.

Dr. Stiler also encouraged me to continue physical therapy. Exercise is helpful in managing the Parkinson's symptoms. Fortunately, I had no problem doing this since I like to exercise.

Over time, I grew more comfortable admitting that I had Parkinson's disease. Other people's responses, however, were a different story. When you tell someone that you have PD, you usually get the sad head bob and the predictable, "I'm sorry." This drives me crazy! Then I will respond, "It's okay. I'm fine." I have found that for me personally, a simple "How are you feeling?" is a much more respectable response. "I'm sorry" makes me feel terrible.

As the disease progressed, I was constantly trying to figure out things to do to help me feel better. Exercise is one of the best ways to slow the progression of PD. Any exercise you enjoy doing is helpful, but there are many news stories that indicate boxing is one of the best exercises for people with PD. I happen to like boxing and have done it in the past. I was happy to start up again to help fight my Parkinson's. I also purchased a stationary bike and would take bike breaks when I worked from home. Some other exercises that I have heard are good for people with PD (or anyone else!) include running, walking, dancing, and swimming. Check with your doctor before starting an exercise program.

Next up were my eating habits. I am not the healthiest of eaters and I never used to eat organic foods. My idea of organic was ordering a pizza from a neighborhood restaurant rather than heating up Ellio's Frozen Pizza. I began trying to reduce or remove processed foods from my diet. Now, I buy organic foods and even organic cleaning products whenever I can. Over the years, I've noticed that reducing processed items and sugar does help me feel better.

Even today, I'm not eating nearly as well as I should, although I am learning to reduce portions and incorporate more healthy items into my meals. But I like what I like and life is short. If I want French fries, I have French fries. If I want a drink, I have a drink.

For me, getting more sleep has been more challenging than eating healthy, especially when I was still working. I used to function well on five to six hours of sleep. With the effects of Parkinson's, I noticed I needed to get six or seven hours of sleep. It can be hard to fit in that extra hour every night.

Getting showered and dressed became an increasingly slower process. It was taking me fifteen minutes to put on and tie my shoes and ninety minutes to shower and get dressed. When you have Parkinson's, you start figuring out simple outfits to put on easily and how long you can go without washing your hair just to save some time. It's a balancing act and it became a challenge to take care of myself.

My walking and balance were alright for a while, but eventually started deteriorating. This brought on the fun task of figuring out which cane works best, which is frustrating but necessary! Unfortunately, for most people with PD, tripping and unstable balance are part of normal life, so a cane becomes an everyday essential item. One of my friends installed handgrips around my house to help me get in and out of doorways. I don't know why doorways became difficult, but they did. Those grips were a blessing.

At work, places I used to easily stroll to for lunch seemed so far away and just traveling back and forth to the office was becoming increasingly harder. The walk to and from the express bus stop during my commute was taking much longer. To get to my building at 1 World Trade Center, I went past the Oculus and the 9/11 Memorial. One day, I was getting frustrated by how long it was taking me, so I sat on a bench and called my boss Matt to ask if he could come down and help me. He did and eventually I was able to get up, hold his arm, follow the blocks in the sidewalk, and walk into the office.

Another example of how amazing Matt was – not just as a boss, but as a person – involved a time when I was having issues with my shoes. Between my terrible walking habits due to Parkinson's, the bunion, and the hammertoe, I had only one pair of shoes I could walk in. My podiatrist recommended that I go to a specialty shoe store in midtown Manhattan. Before Parkinson's, this would not have been a big deal; I simply would have ventured up to the store at lunch and been back in a reasonable amount of time. With PD, I could not do this in the same allotment of time. While I was explaining to Matt about the store, he looked at me and said, "Let's go now." It was 9:30 a.m. Neither of us had any meetings scheduled, so we went. He took me to get shoes because he knew I needed them and could not do it on my own. We traveled there and back by taxi and I did get shoes.

Matt helped me tremendously many times. Eventually, I worked out an arrangement with him to work from home three days a week. As long as I got my work completed, it did not matter where or when I did it. I enjoyed my job, so this made it much easier for me to keep doing it – that is, until I got laid off, along with a bunch of other co-workers, in May 2019. But that is another book…

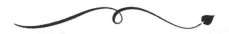

CHAPTER 7
UPS AND DOWNS

As with any illness, living with Parkinson's has its ups and downs, good days, and bad days. I have learned to cope with the negatives and to be extraordinarily grateful for the positives that have come out of this. I have learned a great deal through my Parkinson's story that I feel many others can benefit from, as well, and I'd like to outline some of them here.

Medicine

The Parkinson's medicine is important. This is what should relieve some of your symptoms. You need to be straightforward with your doctor or the medications will not be able to help. Be aware of the following:

- Are side effects impacting you?

- Is the medicine helping?

- How have your symptoms changed since you started taking the medicine?

- If you changed the dosage, what symptoms or side effects changed?

- Is the increased dosage helping?

Exercise

Personally, exercise is just as important in helping me feel good as the medicine. I don't only mean biking on a stationary bike and boxing, which I love. I also mean cleaning the house, doing errands, putting away groceries, working (even if it is volunteering), and staying active. It is not good for anyone, with or without Parkinson's, to sit around all day. Even if you work in an office, be sure to get up and walk around periodically.

If you can exercise, try to do it as early in the day as you can. I find this helps me sleep better because I am not pumping myself up before bedtime.

Stretching

I find that stretching every day, particularly in the morning, helps me walk better. I do abdominal exercises while I stretch, too.

Bad Days

If I am having a bad day, fine! I have my pity party and move on. I try not to let things bring me down for long periods of time.

Falling

I have fallen several times. Sometimes there were nice people around that helped me and sometimes I was alone. Regardless of when and where you fall, you need to pick yourself up and keep moving. It has made me more cautious when I am walking. I tend to look down a lot, but the risk of falling has not stopped me from living my life.

Making Decisions

There may be many people that have – or feel as if they have – input about your health and situation. There are doctors, trainers, family, friends, etc. They mean well, but it's easy to get overwhelmed by decisions to be made as the Parkinson's progresses. It is good to have a sounding board to help you figure out what's right for you, but those decisions are ultimately yours to make. You will be the one living with the results of those decisions.

Nice People

I didn't realize how many nice people there are in the world until I became sick. For example, I cannot begin to tell you how many people have seen me struggling when I walk and asked me if I needed help. One of them, through her upfront approach, also helped me realize I had to get a cane. I was walking to my car from the bus stop, moving slowly. A woman with a cane was walking up the same sidewalk toward me and instinctively asked if I was alright. I responded with a simple, "Yes, thank you." She looked at me for another moment and said, "You do not look alright. Why don't you get yourself a cane?" At that moment, I thought to myself that she was right. It was time to get a cane.

Accepting Help

I used to be one of those people that would try to do everything on my own. I learned, as the PD got worse, to graciously accept help when I needed it. For example, if I needed assistance as I was walking, I would ask to hold the person's arm or hand – whichever worked at the time. I also came to appreciate help with cleaning. I was still working until 2019 and it was hard for me to keep up with work, cleaning my house, and everything I needed to do for my health. A dear friend of mine named Carol cleans houses and she started coming every three or four weeks. We decorated together and had lunch whenever she came. When I got laid off, she did it for free. She still comes today and what I enjoy most is her company.

Keeping Busy

Stay active – physically, mentally, and socially – whether it is virtually or in person.

Modern Conveniences

There are many services and products that help make life easier. Some things I have found to be useful and convenient include:

- Dictating text for messages, emails, documents, and anything else I can when I am not feeling up to typing

- Online shopping for Christmas, birthdays, and everyday items when I am not up to going out

- Ordering my groceries and having them delivered

- Using Click and Ship from the USPS and having my mail carrier take the packages

- Working out at home with exercise equipment that I have, including a stationary bike and a Quiet Punch boxing bag

Feeling Better

Even though I have Parkinson's disease, my life is not only about that. I do other things to make myself feel better. For instance, I visit a wonderful salon to get my hair done and eyelash extensions. I've become friends with the people there, especially the two girls that do my hair. I feel good every time I go and it's a monthly social outing. Another thing I do for myself is to work out with a trainer. I have tried group classes and exercising at home, but neither is as fun as working with a personal trainer. Joe, my trainer, does research to see what will work for me because of the Parkinson's. We box together, which is my favorite thing to do and it makes me excited to go work out. I also stay in touch with friends and family and try to see them as much as I can. In particular, I enjoy going out with my niece Hannah for lunch or shopping and having lunch or dinner with my nephews or cousins. When I'm with them it is fun, but if I need help, they provide it without making me feel disabled.

The most important thing I've learned is that you must do everything in your power to keep living your life. If you don't, Parkinson's disease will take over faster than the Road Runner gets away from Wile E. Coyote. Take control of your life and do what makes you feel good!

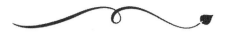

CHAPTER 8
AN UNEXPECTED DETOUR

As time went on, no matter how much I tried to slow the progression of the Parkinson's disease, it seemed like it was advancing faster. I think some of this had to do with me commuting to work. You would think that would help, since it involved exercise and walking, but I noticed when I telecommuted that I was able to move better. Thank goodness for Matt allowing me to have a flexible schedule.

Throughout 2017, I was having even more problems walking and fell at least six times that year. My podiatrist and I tried all different options, including a boot, to help. Finally, in November of 2017, I tore my left Achilles tendon. That pain was terrible and I had no choice but to have surgery in December 2017 right after Christmas, my favorite holiday. Like my mother before me, I love decorating for Christmas, so with the help of family and friends, I still got my Christmas decorations up.

I was not allowed to put weight on my foot for two weeks after the surgery. I didn't want to be totally dependent on other people, so I purchased a knee scooter ahead of time and practiced with it. It was actually easier getting around with the scooter because my left foot was not dragging. I cleared paths and had everything in place for when I would get home. Two of my Great Kills friends came and built a ramp so I would be able to get in and out of the house without facing the stairs. My friends realized that even with the ramp and wheelchair, it would still be difficult for my cousins to get me inside, so one of them arranged for a few FDNY guys to lend a hand. It certainly cheered me up to have four handsome firemen help me get in the house.

The surgery took place at NYU Langone Health Medical Center and was ambulatory, so there was no hospital stay. They could not have been nicer or more efficient. My cousins got me home and the firemen came. I had my scooter and would be in the house recuperating for two weeks. Family members and friends stopped by with food, did my shopping, helped take down my decorations, and assisted me around the house, particularly getting in and out of the shower the first few times. Dr. Scotto, who was down the block, stopped in to check on me. Even for this procedure, I had a good support system from the very beginning, for which I am thankful.

After two weeks, I went to the surgeon for a follow-up appointment. In my head, I was thinking that even though it was not so bad getting around with the scooter, my PD was probably getting worse. Everything was healing well and I could start PT. When I was able to walk, I found that I was not dragging my foot as much. I'm not sure why, but I can only guess that because the Achilles tendon had been weak, it was contributing to me dragging my foot. PD was apparently not the only culprit. It took about a year of physical therapy before I had enough strength to fully exercise, including boxing.

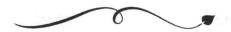

CHAPTER 9
THE DBS SURGERY DECISION

I began talking to Dr. Stiler about DBS surgery again. He explained that it would be better if I had surgery while I was younger because it would improve my quality of life sooner. I started doing some homework to learn more about the surgery and ultimately decided it was time to speak with a surgeon. I had to find out if I were a candidate and how it would work. My doctor recommended Dr. Michael Kaplitt from Weill Cornell Medical Center in Manhattan.

DBS stands for Deep Brain Stimulation surgery. In laymen's terms, I understand it as a way to control Parkinson's by using sensors implanted in your brain that are controlled by batteries. If all goes well, you can reduce your medication and should begin moving better. The detailed definition is: "Deep Brain Stimulation (DBS) is a neurosurgical procedure involving the placement of a medical device called a neurostimulator (sometimes referred to as a brain pacemaker), which sends electrical impulses, through implanted electrodes, to specific targets in the brain (brain nuclei) for the treatment of movement disorders, including Parkinson's disease, essential tremor, and dystonia."

Initially, I put it out of my mind because my medicine was working and I was moving as well as could be expected. Honestly, I did not like the idea of equipment in my body. I was doing alright, so I would stick to that course of action for the time being. Surgery would be my last choice if things got worse.

I finally knew it was time to seriously consider surgery when my friends and I went to Madison Square Garden to see Elton John and I voluntarily asked for a wheelchair. My friends almost fainted and I felt like I was losing my fight with PD.

One big mistake I made was thinking that DBS surgery was a last resort – my ace in the hole. In fact, it should be considered as soon as you are eligible, pending a discussion with your doctor. It is a quality-of-life improvement, not a cure, and will not save your life.

Before you can decide if you want to have DBS surgery, you need to find out if you're a candidate. That determination may vary for each person, depending upon a range of criteria such as their symptoms, their physician's evaluation, etc. I made an appointment for May 22, 2019 and Greta, Erin, and Dorothea would be coming with me. An ironic thing happened on my journey before this appointment. A decision came from upper management at Moody's that Matt had to lay off me and other employees. I was called into his office and he had to read a speech that the HR department had written. The speech was not something Matt would ever say to me. He was crying; I was crying. I got laid off from Moody's on May 21. I was nervous enough going to the surgeon and deciding whether to have this life-altering surgery, but now I also had no job. I put that out of my mind, made sure my health insurance was in order, and prepared myself for the next day's meeting with the surgeon.

The four of us headed to Manhattan for my appointment with the surgeon and his nurse practitioner. Greta was asking questions, Erin was taking notes, and I was listening. Dr. Kaplitt and Kristin, the nurse practitioner, asked a lot of questions and gave us a lot of information. I knew by the end of the appointment that I was a candidate for the DBS surgery. Now I had to decide if I would do it and then go for an MRI. After the appointment, we came back to Staten Island for lunch, cocktails, and a discussion that ended with me deciding to have the surgery. Greta, Erin, and Dorothea are three of the closest people in my life. I have no problem putting my life in their hands and it was fitting that they were the ones with me to make this decision.

We gathered lots of important information about the surgery during this meeting. The surgeon I met with performs DBS in two separate surgeries. The first one is to put the sensors in your brain, one on either side. You are awake during this because you need to do exercises with the neurologist during the procedure. Only local anesthesia is used.

The second surgery is done about a week later, to run wires and implant the batteries for the sensors. This procedure was intended to address tremors, stiffness, cramping in my foot, and possibly my freezing gait issues. It would not directly help with walking and balance, but by minimizing these other symptoms, I would be able to exercise better and improve my walking and balance as a result.

Once I decided that I wanted to move ahead, I had to go for two tests. The first was a psych test to evaluate logic and memory. It was long but kind of fun. The second was an hour-long MRI that was used to determine where the sensors would go. After these were done, the surgeon had the information needed to officially determine whether I was truly a candidate.

Based on the information my doctors and surgeon had provided, the surgery seemed as if it would be largely successful. Other people's symptoms had been improved, thus improving their quality of life. I spoke to a few who had the surgery and felt reassured that it helped them lead better lives.

At last, I was deemed a candidate for the DBS surgery and I made the decision to move forward. My first surgery was scheduled for September 24, 2019.

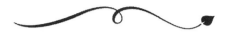

CHAPTER 10
GETTING READY FOR DBS

If you are planning on having DBS, your doctor should give you instructions on how to prepare for the surgeries. Follow them! If you have any questions, do not hesitate to call your doctor and ask them. Remember…this is brain surgery!

The items below are additional things I did that I found helpful in getting ready.

Clothes

When you come home after the first surgery, there will be stitches and staples in your head. Have clothes set aside, especially shirts, that are easy to put on.

For women, after the second surgery, you probably will not be able to put on a bra because of the stitches and staples for the batteries. I stocked up on tank tops and camisoles to double-layer under comfortable shirts.

Necessities

I live on my own and stupidly thought I would be up and taking care of myself within a day of each surgery. Both of my surgeries were on Tuesdays. Each time, I did not feel well enough to take care of myself until Friday. Especially after the first surgery, I was tired! Stock up on foods, medicines, etc. before the first surgery, whether they are for you or whomever lives with you.

Company

If you live alone, be sure to have someone stay with you for a night or two, particularly after the first surgery.

Keep Busy

Leading up to the first surgery, I was quite nervous. The best advice I got from a friend was to stay busy, so I kept myself occupied by writing a blog about the surgery and doing other things. I am passing this advice on to you, too. Keep busy.

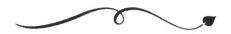

CHAPTER 11
DBS, PART ONE

The day of the first surgery arrived. I had to be at the hospital at 5:30 a.m. Who does anything at that hour? My stepson Mike and I were in Manhattan in plenty of time. I had my surgery done at Weill Cornell Presbyterian Hospital by Dr. Michael Kaplitt. He was excellent and, first and foremost, all the nurses were wonderful. Each one was nicer than the next and could not be more helpful. There was one woman, who I believe was a physician assistant, who worked with Dr. Kaplitt. She was terrific at explaining everything that was going to happen.

From this point on, I am going to be brutally honest about what the surgery involves and what the pain felt like to me.

Before the surgery started, I needed to change into the hospital scrubs. I had no medicine or food in me and was moving slower than usual. I didn't want my stepson to help because I'm stubborn and thought I could do it myself. Eventually, I must have been moving too slowly for things to stay on schedule so a nurse came in to help.

As I was sitting in the pre-surgery room with Mike, waiting for the next step, it dawned on me that in a blog I had read about the surgery, this was the hardest part – having the frame put on. It is funny how you put some things out of your mind, but it was too late now to back out.

The metal frame was placed onto my head. For it to stay in position, four screws needed to be inserted: two in the forehead and two in the back of the head. The most unpleasant part was the numbing needles shoved into my head before they put the screws in place. After the frame was on, I felt like Darth Vader! My poor stepson was watching this entire procedure, but it was somewhat calming for me to have him there.

Next came a CT scan. I was taken to a room where I laid down and my head was snapped in place with the frame on before I went into the machine for the CT scan. So far, this was easy compared to what lay ahead.

Next it was on to the operating room. Throughout the procedure, the most difficult part of this surgery was not being in control of the situation. Your head is locked in this device and you cannot do anything. I understood this was necessary, but for me, there was a feeling of panic that came along with this immobility.

During the surgery, the doctor started on one side and then moved to the other side. Since my Parkinson's was impacting both sides of my body, he was working on both sides of my brain during one surgery. I'm glad he did it that way because I don't know whether I could have gone through this twice knowing how it worked.

The local anesthesia is like when you go to a dentist and they give you Novocaine shots; the injections hurt more than the work being done. For DBS surgery, you are essentially having needles shoved into your head, which, as could be expected, is not the most pleasant experience. Luckily, you cannot feel anything once the numbing shots take effect. However, you do still hear the drill. It is loud.

Once they drilled the opening, they put the sensor inside and tested it. This is to set the sensor to the maximum stimulus you can take and it is done so that when programming starts, they know what you can withstand. In my case, my eye and lip started twitching when the stimulus was too much. I am currently not programmed near the max.

After the doctor puts the sensor in place, you next do a series of tests with the neurologist. This is the whole purpose of being awake through this surgery. The neurologist had me open and close my hand and grip his hand. All my tests went well and when they were finished, the doctor closed the wounds. The most uncomfortable part about this was not the stitches, but the staples. Having something that sounds like a staple gun working on your head is a bit unnerving.

They moved on to the other side of my head and again, the tests went well. Thankfully, after the second side was done and the closing was finished, the frame came off. There was a slight complication with one of my screws and the doctor had to put in a staple after they removed the frame. Although it was upsetting, I kept my composure through the whole surgery because I knew I had to. When it was over, I finally started crying. I guess my emotions got the best of me and it was very tough.

After the surgery was completed and the frame taken off my head, I was brought into the recovery room, still crying from the overwhelming emotions. I had my own nurse and there were other people around to help. They were not telling me to calm down, just trying to distract me. It worked and I was finally able to calm down.

After being in surgery for six hours, I had to use the restroom. One of the nurses came over with a bedpan and I laughed. I have a very shy bladder and cannot pee unless no one is watching and I'm in the regular position. As you can imagine, the bedpan experience did not go very well, so I waited for my room to be ready before trying again. While in recovery, I also got hungry and had to wait for my Parkinson's pills. Mike went to Starbucks and brought me back two of my favorites – some pumpkin bread and a chocolate chip cookie. He's awesome.

The point of all this is that, once I went to recovery, my normal bodily cravings kicked in. I am guessing it was because I was no longer under anesthesia. I was a little tired, but that was it. The surgery began at 11 a.m. and I was in recovery and then taken to a room by 4 p.m. Not too bad.

Although I had a private room, the annoying thing about being in a hospital overnight is all the poking and prodding and checking that needs to be done. They check your vitals every couple of hours, so you don't get any sleep when you really need it. At one point, I asked the poor nurse, "How long will it be before you come back?"

When I woke up on Wednesday morning, I decided that nobody was going to tell me how to take my pills or how to take care of myself. I had been doing it for years. My nurse came in and I informed him, "I am taking my pills and getting out of this bed because with the Parkinson's, lying around is not good for me." He helped me up and when my doctor arrived to check on me, everything went well and I was able to go home. I sat waiting for my stepson to return for me and before I left,

I apologized to my nurse. He told me not to worry about it, because he would have done the same thing.

When I got home and started my regular cadence of medication and supplements, I couldn't keep my eyes open. Since I'd had no sleep Monday after a major surgery, I was wiped out. I was taken aback by how tired I was.

On Thursday, I started getting black and blue marks on my face, as they told me might happen. I pretty much looked like I went a few rounds with my trainers if they were to hit me back. I had to put ice packs on my face and sit up straight to manage the swelling. Beginning that day, I was sleeping, sitting up straight, and showering every night. I was starting to feel better.

Mike stayed until Friday, constantly checking on me and asking if I needed anything. I required this level of attention and care that first week. As I continued to feel better, other family members and friends came to check in on me, also.

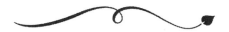

CHAPTER 12
DBS, PART TWO, TAKE ONE

My next surgery was scheduled for Tuesday, October 8. My neurosurgeon told me this surgery would be easier. It was only an hour-long procedure and I would be asleep for the whole thing, but it didn't seem like it would be easy to me. I hate going under anesthesia and my imagination was getting the best of me about how big the wires and the batteries implanted into my body would be. It probably would have been better if they had shown them to me ahead of time. I've always said if something is left to my imagination, I will imagine the worst.

One thing I had not done up until that point was to figure out what else I could expect to change in response to the surgery. For example, my physical therapy would change. I have herniated discs in my neck and my therapist would work on my neck once a week. However, the surgery would involve inserting wires going down either side of my neck, so my therapist would need to figure out a new approach to working on those discs. This was not necessarily an earth-shattering realization, but I knew it was a conscious change that must take place for me to maintain my overall health. I needed to remember to reach out to my physical therapist to make him aware of this lifestyle change. I tried to document anyone else I needed to reach out to for information. This is something you should try to do before the surgery if possible. You want to make sure you understand what else may be impacted by this surgery so you can prepare and ask the appropriate questions from the right people.

In between surgeries, it became difficult to be at home on my own much of the time. That was the mental challenge of dealing with this surgery. I had far too much time on my hands to think and tried to keep myself busy so I would not dwell on the upcoming surgery. I used some of my spare time to document the surgery in my blog, but there's only so much you can do with staples and stiches in your head. I needed to remember I was undergoing this surgery because it was my best chance to have a good quality of life. I had made the decision to go forward and now I had to stay focused.

Another friend of mine sent me an email and told me that I had courage for going through this and would be stronger when it was over. This helped me. Remembering words of encouragement from family and friends was important for getting me through the lonely times.

The morning of October 8 started out alright. My friend Kristin was accompanying me for this second phase of my surgery. We had to be at the hospital at 8:45 a.m. and arrived ten minutes early. I got ready for the surgery and was brought to the operating room. This first part of the surgery required general anesthesia and just as they started the procedure, they had to stop because my blood pressure went high and my heart rate went low. I had a bad reaction to some of the anesthesia medication and phase two of the DBS procedure did not happen that day. The doctors were concerned about my heart and I was upset that the DBS surgery could not be completed yet.

That visit turned into a hospital stay all the way through Friday. The doctors ran many different heart tests to check that I was in healthy and stable condition. Those days in the hospital were a scary week for me. I amazed myself at how well I was taking the various ups and downs and emotional stress of the situation. Part of the reason I was able to handle it so well was the staff at Weill Cornell Presbyterian Hospital. First I was in ICU and then I was moved to the neurosurgery step down unit. All the nurses, nurse's aides, physician assistants, and doctors were very attentive, caring, and helpful. You could not ask for better people to take care of you. Dr. Kaplitt always made me feel comfortable and calm and he made sure things got done. Finally, on Friday I had a cardiac CAT scan that showed I had no blockages. I was cleared to go home and the second DBS surgery was rescheduled for Tuesday, October 15. I was excited and so were my nurses and PA.

I couldn't help but wonder if I would be able to finish the DBS surgery so that I could move forward and hopefully improve my quality of life from the Parkinson's. I had great faith in Dr. Kaplitt and his team, which is what kept me motivated to go back the following Tuesday.

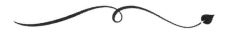

CHAPTER 13
DBS, PART TWO, TAKE TWO

Annmarie and Tommie took me for my rescheduled surgery. The second time worked like a charm and everything went as planned.

What happened the previous week was further explained to me. This was helpful, but I was still a bit nervous and when I was wheeled into the surgery room, I broke down a bit. The staff could not have been more accommodating to help me feel better. They had me lay down and get a sedative to take the edge off, which really helped. The surgery went on for about one and a half hours, everything went smoothly, and I woke up with no problems. Due to the placement of the batteries, I was a little sore around my collarbone and, of course, there were stitches in my head but overall, this second surgery was not half as bad as I thought it would be.

A few days later, other than being sore, I felt alright. I slept a lot after both surgeries; in fact, I slept nearly twenty-eight hours in three days. With all the staples and stitches, it felt kind of stiff to move, but I got a little better each day.

I was excited to start the process of turning on the devices, but even more excited by then to get all the stitches and staples removed. I had never had so many staples in my body and it was not particularly fun. My hair needed a lot of work from my hairdressers, too. Between the doctor shaving my head, the rubber bands they put in for the surgery (which had to be to cut out), and all the blood and gross stuff that gets in your hair, it was a mess! I had cut my hair shorter before the surgery, but not short enough. That was honestly the least of my concerns, but I do feel it's something to think of if you are considering the surgery. It's always amazing how the stuff you think is important at one point, like your hair, becomes inconsequential when there are staples in your head.

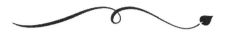

CHAPTER 14
TURNING ON THE DEVICES

O ctober 24 was the big day. The devices were to be turned on and we would see if the surgery worked, but first, the stitches and staples needed to come out. I was concerned that if it had been so painful to put them in, how they could be taken out without hurting. I'm happy to say that they were removed pain-free. I was talking to Kristin, the nurse practitioner, and Erin and before I knew it, the stitches were all removed. Now I would be able to wash and condition my hair without stitches or staples getting in the way. It had been a month of dealing with this. It is the little things in life you miss when you don't have them anymore.

I was a bit worried about turning on the devices. All sorts of questions were running through my head. What if it did not work? What if something is wrong? There were two things keeping me calm. One was my friend by my side. The other was that both sensors were tested during the first surgery once they were placed in my head. This was the surgery for which I was awake and had to test with the neurologist. I knew the sensors worked.

Before the programming session could begin, the vendor representative from Abbott, the company that makes my devices, needed to give me a lesson on how they worked. The primary device he went over with me was the patient controller. On this controller, the person doing the programming for the sensors can set up ranges for me to control. Awesome!

Kristin started programming and suddenly, my shaking calmed down. It was nothing short of amazing. Everything I did to get to this point was worth it. Matt, who was supporting me through this whole endeavor, had told me the scary parts were behind me. Now was the phase of excitement, opportunity, and hard work. He was right. I tried to let my body tell me what it was feeling and not control the situations with my brain. Eventually, we got into a good rhythm and I was able to tell Kristin what felt alright and what did not. It is important to be honest with whomever does your programming to get the most out of it. I would say, "That doesn't feel right." She would ask why and sometimes I would simply say, "I don't know. It just doesn't."

We got both sides of my brain initially programmed, then we took a break. I took my Parkinson's and essential tremors medicines and after about thirty minutes, we met again. We made some final adjustments and that was it. Leaving the office that day, I had the patient controller in hand, was not shaking much, and was moving much better. The controller would allow me to adjust preset ranges up or down as needed. For the time being, we were leaving my medicine doses as they were.

The first three days were incredible. I felt like I had gone back in time to when I first started getting sick. I was not as stiff, my tremors were minimal, and I felt good. In the event program from the 2019 Drive Away Parkinson's golf outing I organized, I had written the following: "Fighting Parkinson's can be compared to playing defense in the National Football

League. When you first get a diagnosis that you have Parkinson's disease, it is the equivalent of having the offense pinned inside their five-yard line. You start trying a combination of medicine and exercise to keep Parkinson's on its side of the field for as long as possible. While medicine is necessary, exercise and a day-to-day routine that keeps you moving are the keys to holding back Parkinson's. Eventually, it will cross the fifty-yard line and you need different plays to fight it. This is the next step for me, with the hopes of pushing Parkinson's back to its side of the field."

The DBS surgery has pushed Parkinson's back better than I could have hoped. I noticed many changes after the initial programming session, including the following:

- I was not as stiff as I was; not even close.

- My walking improved. I still followed the blocks in the sidewalk, but it was easier, I didn't need a cane, and I could talk when I walked. I was also moving both arms when I walked, which was something I had not done in years.

- My cousin came with me for my test drive so I could start driving again. He is a retired Marine, so I figured if something went wrong, he would know what to do. It went well and I was back to my old self.

- My tremors were minimal.

I had to continue exercising and stretching, but I still needed time to heal from the surgeries. Additionally, there was more programming to be done, although after just one programming session, I was excited and hopeful.

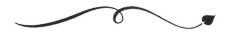

CHAPTER 15
FOLLOW-UP PROGRAMMING

A little of my shaking came back by the following Tuesday, so when I called the doctor's office, Kristin approved me upping the impulses using the patient controller. I cannot feel anything when I do this but my movements got better, so I knew it worked.

I learned to determine which shaking came from essential tremors versus Parkinson's. The surgery is meant to help PD, although mine seems to have also reduced my essential tremors. Below are some initial observations:

- My head was still tender where the staples and stitches were. This is normal and can take up to three months to heal.

- Over the weekend, I was doing stuff around the house, such as laundry. I could not believe how fast I could fold the clothes. It had been years since I did laundry at a normal pace.

- I drove with my cousin Tommy and that went well. In fact, we drove and then walked.

- I got the okay to ride my stationary bike. The first time, I did it for ten minutes and it felt good.

These things may not seem like such a big deal to you, but when you go for a long period of time moving at a snail's pace, returning close to normal while you have a non-curable disease is pretty amazing. For the first time in a long time, I was looking forward to the future. Each day, I noticed something else that had improved and we had not even done the second round of programming yet. Some of these new improvements included:

- My upper lip was not shaking.

- Handwriting in script was easier to do and much more legible. I still take notes and make lists and now I can read them again.

- Tying my shoes was back to normal.

- Typing on my phone and laptop was easier and faster.

- Overall, getting dressed was easier. I used to dread putting on a bra and shirt, but now it was better than it had been in years.

- I was not using a cane anymore

- I was having a problem before the surgery with drooling, but it stopped after the device was turned on.

- I could open bottles again.

- I could once again cut my own food.

- I was back to talking with my hands and speaking fast. Whether that is a good thing or not, the fact that I can do it again is great!

- My walking continued to improve and I am less stiff when I walk. I walked by myself to a diner around the corner to get lunch. Other than going to my doctor's office on the corner, I could not remember the last time I had walked anywhere alone.

To help my body to heal from the surgeries, I did the following:

- My sleeping habits were terrible prior to the surgeries and I would only get five to six hours of sleep a night. After the surgeries, I made a point of getting seven to eight hours of sleep.

- My eating habits were not much better than my sleeping habits prior to surgery. Afterwards, I tried to eat as healthy as I could, with everything in moderation. I learned that most people gain five to ten pounds after the surgery, but I am not sure why. Healthy eating is important.

- I stopped drinking prior to the surgeries and while I was healing, I kept it to just an occasional drink from time to time.

All these lifestyle changes are small when you see what the DBS surgery is giving back in exchange.

Once I maxed out the ranges on the patient controller, I needed to go back to the surgeon's office in Manhattan on November 14 to do more programming and testing. This time,

I commuted on my own from Staten Island. I was able to walk easier and it felt good to be out and about.

When we started the session that day, the program I had been using was saved as a backup, so I could go back to it if I needed to with my patient controller. We tested a mix of other programs, including one that did not work nearly as well, so we deleted it. By the end of the session, we found a combination that worked and I felt great. I even traveled downtown in the city to visit friends.

During that session, I also asked how I would know when my batteries, which last four to five years, must be changed. I was told that the controller will alert me and then I would schedule a visit to have them replaced.

It is quite fascinating how my body reacts to the electric stimulation. If it is turned off, you can see my hands and body shake from the tremors, my face does not show much expression, and all my other symptoms come back. When the stimulation is on and working, I can feel my body calm down. I stop shaking and move better. It's like turning back time to when I first got sick but was still able to move alright. It is incredible and I am beyond happy with the results of the DBS surgery so far. I still have work to do, but I don't mind.

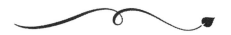

CHAPTER 16
LIFE AFTER DBS SURGERY

While I was healing and going for programming sessions, the 2019 holidays snuck up on us. The holiday season is my favorite time of year. Yes, I believe it is an entire season rather than just a day. I started decorating Thanksgiving weekend. Immediately, I noticed I was able to do things twice as fast as before the surgery – unwrapping ornaments, putting out my villages, taking stuff in and out of the boxes, etc. I was able to get my house fully decorated, wrap all the gifts, and mail the cards.

For our annual Girls Christmas, my friends and I traditionally rotate the houses where it is held. In 2019, after the surgery, I was able to have it at my house on December 14. Thanks to my ability to move better, I was able to do all the cooking, shopping, and setting the table without a problem in preparation for the day. We shared many laughs, drank champagne, and opened presents; the day was a big success!

In early January 2020, I received the good news that all my doctors agreed I was doing great. Kristin, the nurse practitioner, said that we were finished programming for the time being. I could start boxing again and continue to live my life. I would come in for a follow-up appointment about three months later.

In January, I also went back to physical therapy. It was about three months after the first surgery and as it turns out, Vinny could no longer work on my neck. This was because the leads connecting the sensors in my brain to the batteries near my collarbone go behind my ears and down by my neck and shoulders, which is right where he used to work on me. No more massages or stimulation by anyone or anything. When I stop and think about this, it is a small price to pay for how good I feel. Plan B for my neck is a pillow I found on Amazon that is designed to help with neck pain and it does work! At PT, I rode the stationary bike and did leg exercises. As much as I don't particularly enjoy those, they're needed to improve my balance and walking, so I just put on my music and did what I needed to do.

One of the best things that happened in January was that I started boxing again. It's a good exercise for anyone, but is especially helpful for people with Parkinson's disease. I started with my Quiet Punch bag at home and my punches were harder. Later in the week, I boxed with my trainer Joe, who said my punches were better than they had ever been.

I would use the arm bike at PT to loosen up before boxing. The first time I did it after the surgery was shocking to me. Prior to the surgery, using the bike on a tension of 2.5 for six minutes was a challenge. It felt like I was moving a heavy weight and I was awfully slow. On this particular day, the bike was set at 3.0 for ten minutes and I pedaled faster than I was ever able to.

I would also do balance and hand/eye coordination exercises, which included playing catch, standing on one foot and catching the ball. I had not been able to balance on one foot before, but now I could. It was encouraging to see progress.

Vinny told me to be patient and take things slow and steady – but I'm not very good at being patient.

I went into the city for a programming session in February. It was more like a tune-up. I call it that because we did not need to change any of the programs much; it was more about adding ranges for me to adjust the programs on my own if symptoms come back. After the doctor's appointment, I had lunch downtown with a friend. The doctor's office is uptown and I was able to get around the city on my own by walking and taking a cab, which felt great. I am very independent already, and the more independence I get back, the better I feel.

Since the surgery, I've noticed it has been easier to brush, floss, and rinse my teeth with Listerine. I had to go to the dental hygienist for a teeth cleaning and she was done so fast, I was surprised. She was pleased with the improvement in my dental care and so was I. Now I don't have to dread the cleaning anymore! I also spoke with the dentist and he was amazed at how well the surgery worked. He mentioned that in the past, my tremors were so bad that it was hard to work on me. This time, he was done in about twenty minutes. I was two for two with good dentist appointments.

Around this time, I had been asked to participate in a podcast called "This Is Your Brain with Dr. Phil Stieg." The podcast would be a conversation with Dr. Phil Stieg, Dr. Michael Kaplitt, and me. The topic, of course, was Parkinson's disease and DBS surgery. We recorded the podcast in early March and I enjoyed doing it tremendously. We spoke for over an hour. Later in the year, when it was released, it would end up being two podcasts instead of just one.

In March, I attended a charity event and what happened there falls into the "this was meant to be" category. Guests were able to sit wherever they pleased, so Ginny, Mike, and I picked a table with a nice family. We had a great time all night and I even won the basket they had donated. At the end of the night, I gave the husband one of the cards for my golf outing. He shared that his wife had Parkinson's. I asked her if she had researched DBS surgery, but she admitted she was not ready for that yet. That was my position not too long ago. Everything happens for a reason.

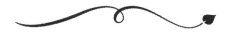

CHAPTER 17
THE 2020 PANDEMIC IMPACT

As I write this, we are in the middle of the global COVID-19 pandemic, which has kept most of us quarantined in our homes for weeks at a time. For someone like me, it's important to keep moving and exercising. I have been unable to attend PT during this time, although I can still go out for walks if the weather is nice.

During the pandemic, I started walking around the neighborhood. There's a post office about seven or eight blocks away that I walk to, and on the way home, I stop at the deli to grab a sandwich for lunch and then finish my walk. I listen to music and it feels wonderful. I still need to improve my walking because I'm leaning too much to my right side. I've been doing that for so long, it's going to take me a while to break the habit.

It is one thing to walk around my house or backyard where I am comfortable. It is another thing to walk on different sidewalks, up and down hills, etc. My first long walk, post-surgery, was 3,800 steps and the second was 2,900 steps. Each time, I felt like I was walking almost normally – slowly, but with better form. I have been trying to go for at least one long walk per week, depending on the weather. Recently during quarantine, I walked 4,600 steps, or about 1.5 miles. My feet hurt a bit and my legs were a little tired, but I did it without a cane and was quite proud of myself.

I had a doctor's appointment with my neurologist via phone call since the pandemic prevents in-person visits. It was strange but served its purpose, although it would have been much harder had I not gone through with the DBS surgery.

Thankfully, I am now doing well. I have been holding steady in the ranges for the stimulus, with no shaking or stiffness. I have settled into a very productive exercise routine at home. Most mornings, I stretch, do ab exercises, and recently added a few planks. I do cardio using the stationary bike two days a week and box two days a week, as well. Besides helping my Parkinson's, these activities also help my emotional well-being.

From a DBS standpoint, the levels on my patient controller device are set for now. Prior to the surgery, I was told my Parkinson's would be managed with a combination of the DBS and my medicine. The hope was that we would eventually reduce the amount of medicine, which we did. I am down to taking two Ropinirole pills (Parkinson's medicine); at one point, I was taking four pills. I am still taking Azilect for the Parkinson's and for the essential tremors, I was able to cut the dosage of the Propranolol in half and eliminate one Primidone pill.

Mike has told me I look great, like I did before Parkinson's hit, and how happy and proud of me he is. That is one of the nicest compliments I have ever received.

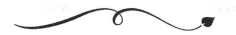

CHAPTER 18
TAKING ACTION

O nce I had taken control of my own Parkinson's disease, I decided I needed to be more involved in helping to find a cure. I had helped run charity golf outings in the past, so I thought a golf outing would be a good way to raise money to donate to Parkinson's research. I asked a friend if he would help run a golf outing for PD. He said yes and from that point on, it was full speed ahead.

My nephew Peter helped me come up with the name for a nonprofit. Since the primary fundraising event would be a golf outing, we focused on the word "drive." And so, Drive Away Parkinson's (DAP) was created.

A gentleman I worked with at Moody's, who is a software engineer as well as a first-class artist, brainstormed with me. We came up with the idea for the logo and he brought it to life. I still have the original drawing hanging in my home office. I absolutely love our logo!

With our name decided and the logo designed, I knew we had to create the non-profit company. It needed to be a 501(c)(3) so people could write off their donations, so I went to a lawyer and we drafted the necessary paperwork. The IRS stamped the approval letter for the 501(c)(3) with the date of September 14, 2016. That would have been my mom's 75th birthday. To me, this was a sign of her approval for what I was doing.

I created a board for the company, made up of family and friends. The initial board included fifteen members, with a mix of people from my life's journey so far. It is made up of two cousins, five Great Kills friends, three friends from work, three North Shore friends, and my physical therapist. We held our first meeting at a friend's restaurant, where the board members got to know each other and started planning our first golf outing.

While I was establishing Drive Away Parkinson's and the golf outing, I was also taking golf lessons with the pro at the Richmond County Country Club (RCCC). This is a private club with a beautiful golf course and ballroom. I was not a member, although my physical therapist was and he arranged for me to take lessons. The pro and I hit it off and he was a nice guy. Aside from being a great golfer, he played fantasy football, which I also did and could talk about all day. We both liked Matchbox 20, so he would play their music during my lessons. This helped me focus.

One day, we were talking about the golf outing that I was planning and that it would be the first one. The pro asked if I would consider hosting the outing at the RCCC, explaining that non-member outings take place on Mondays. I was excited to hear about this option and jumped at the opportunity. Having my outing at this exclusive golf club would help me bring in players, since people are only allowed to golf there if they are a member or participating in an outing. There was only one Monday available for an outing at the RCCC; all the rest were booked. Our outing is now planned annually on the third Monday in July.

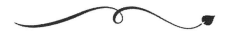

CHAPTER 19
DAP FUNDRAISING

I am a project manager by training and have helped run other golf outings in the past. Planning and executing a successful golf outing was in my wheelhouse.

A decision had to be made regarding where the money we raised would go. We researched Parkinson's organizations, including one in Staten Island. The work being done by the Michael J. Fox Foundation was most impressive to us. Their current slogan is "Here. Until Parkinson's isn't." I appreciate their urgency and dedication in finding a cure. We have been working with this foundation since the beginning and 100% of the money we raise for them goes to Parkinson's research.

I booked the golf course plus the ballroom for the dinner afterwards. I knew I wanted to make it a festive atmosphere. After a long day of golfing, you must keep people engaged with an exciting dinner, so we hired a DJ. I wanted balloon centerpieces so they would not be in the way of people talking to each other. I got a recommendation to visit a local shop called Chocolate Fantasy. Remember my life philosophy that everything happens for a reason? Well, I met the owner and told her about my fundraiser and that I had Parkinson's. As it turns out, her dad also had Parkinson's and passed away. She and I have been friends ever since that first meeting. She is a generous, wonderful woman.

Next on the list was bringing in sponsors, golfers, and raffle gifts. The entire board helped. For our inaugural event, we were all learning how to do things – for example, contacting companies for raffle donations. There is something different you need to do for each request. Over the years, we have learned that the most generous corporate sponsors are the NY Giants and Jets and they always give a signed football. This is particularly exciting to me since football is my favorite sport to watch.

We did well gathering local and corporate sponsors for our first golf outing. I have generous friends who are local business owners and they support my fight against Parkinson's disease year after year. I also have many family and friends that donate raffle baskets, money, and time to make the events successful. I will never be able to thank them enough.

Over the first three years, we have managed to have about ninety-five golfers at each outing, in large part due to my group of Great Kills friends. At least half of the golfers are friends I have had for forty-plus years. The rest of the golfers include friends from Moody's, high school, and others I've met over the years, plus people who want the opportunity to golf at the Richmond County Country Club. Each year, we get one or two new foursomes of people that want to golf there. My goal for the next outing is to reach one hundred golfers.

Even though many people told me I should keep the post-outing dinner moving and as brief as possible because it comes at the end of a long day, my thinking was different. The golfers in the first year were not teeing off until 12:00 p.m. (we've moved it to 11:00 since then). It is a long day, but they are golfing, not working. I wanted a party afterward and that is how I planned it. We had a DJ, beautiful centerpieces, great food, raffles, silent auction items, a 50/50 raffle, and other prizes, all to fit within a three-hour event. The project manager in me kicked in and I laid out the day, hour by hour, before reviewing the plan with the board, golf course, and banquet manager. I was watching the weather forecast starting twenty-five days out. That is something I cannot control, which is maddening!

The day of the first golf outing finally arrived. My brother and niece were staying with me and I had to be at the golf course early to meet the board and greet people. A friend picked me up and as soon as we pulled into the parking lot, the skies opened up. It was a monsoon! I remained amazingly calm. My pro was keeping an eye on the storm and kept telling me it would pass. My friend looked at me and asked if we should call it off. This was at 11:20 a.m. My reply was, "Absolutely not." Sure enough, before tee time, the sun came out and it was a beautiful, temperate day. The course dried up and it was perfect! By the way, this monsoon weather would also happen the second year and it rained late in the afternoon of the third year.

We had ninety golfers and about one hundred twenty-eight people, including most of the golfers, at the dinner. For our first outing, it went extremely well. One friend declared it "outstanding." I had been waiting for a compliment like that for years! I received many nice remarks about how great the outing was and how kind the people on the board were, who were doing much of the work along with the staff at the country club. Over the years, we have compiled a list of lessons learned after each outing and fine-tuned it for the next year. We raised $15,000 that first year and I could not have been happier.

We were donating this money to the Michael J. Fox Foundation to be used for Parkinson's research. I wasn't sure how this worked and did not want to mail a $15,000 check – never thinking I could send it to them electronically. I called their office in Manhattan and asked if a few board members and I could bring the check to them. They were very nice and said yes. We went to the office and they gave us a tour, where we took some pictures with them. I didn't know until I went to an appreciation dinner the next year that this was not normal operating procedure. Since I had called and asked, they accommodated me. That is a class act!

In our second year of operation, a friend who lived in Manhattan offered to change a Chili Cook-Off he has with friends into a fundraiser for Drive Away Parkinson's. The couple hosting had a beautiful apartment with more than enough room to hold this event and it turned out to be quite fun. We have had this fundraiser for the last two years and have raised approximately $2,000 each year. I appreciate the generosity of the hosts and their friends.

Since the inception of Drive Away Parkinson's, we have donated $56,000 to the Michael J. Fox Foundation to be used for Parkinson's research.

And my journey continues.

THE FIRST BOARD OF DRIVE AWAY PARKINSONS

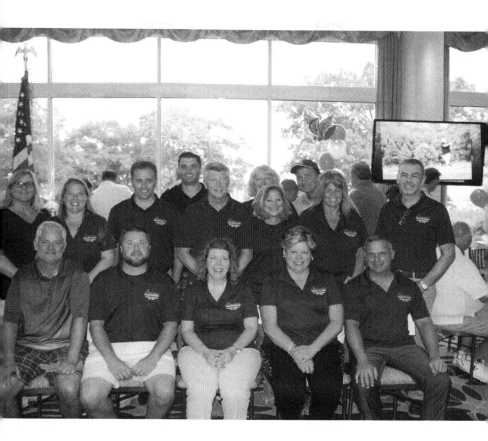

Front Row – Ben Hill, Steve Sandberg, Me, Annmarie Goodheart, Vinny Puccio

Middle Row – Kristin Strandberg, Camille Sandberg, Brice Palmer, Matt Barton, Dorothea Zando, Greta Barton, Pat O'Sullivan

Back Row – Brian Armocida, Erin Reardon, Paul Sneddon

Missing – Diana DiLeo

EPILOGUE

As of the writing of this book, I am in good health. I'm trying to eat healthy and exercise as much as I can. I have gone six months without adjusting the patient controller. If I need to, I can, but for now I am good. I am back in the gym working out with Joe and feeling better than I have in years.

If you have Parkinson's and your doctor recommends DBS surgery, you should consider it! My neurologist initially recommended this years ago. I thought it was my last resort rather than a way to improve my quality of life. I was so wrong. It took many people convincing me that I should at least find out if I was eligible for the surgery before I finally talked to the surgeon. I am glad I did.

Made in the USA
Coppell, TX
29 August 2021